FROM

STRENGTH

TO

STRENGTH

AN OSTEOPATH'S APPROACH TO HEALTH

British Library cataloguing-in-publication data. A catalogue record for this book is available from the British Library.

First Published in Great Britain, 1993 by
The Boxmoor Osteopathic Press
Hemel Hempstead.

Practice details:

THE
BOXMOOR OSTEOPATHIC
PRACTICE

Communications

Tel: 01442 255610

Fax: 01442 255610

Practice address

9 Northridge Way
Boxmoor
Hemel Hempstead
Herts
HP1 2AE

BOXMOOR PRACTICE
CONSULTATION TIMES

We provide a full 7 day service, based on the assumption that a bad back or an injury is a problem no matter whatever time it arises. This service will provide you with cover seven days a week. Appointments may be arranged by telephone, which is generally manned over the full 24 hours.

Home visits are also made to patients who are unable to travel (fee available on request).

PRACTICE RULE

A general rule which I try to follow when treating any injury is that suggested by Andrew Taylor Still the founder of Osteopathy:

"Find it, fix it, and leave it alone."

EDUCATIONAL TALKS

For any interested groups educational talks on Osteopathy are available on request.

DIRECTIONS TO:

THE BOXMOOR OSTEOPATHIC PRACTICE

M1 North

M1 South

M1 Jn. 8

A414

HEMEL HEMPSTEAD
TOWN CENTRE

Tesco superstore
Jarman's fields

A4146
to
LEIGHTON
BUZZARD

Magic
Roundabout

River Gade

Station Road

to KINGS LANGLEY

to M25 Jn. 20

A4251 (Was A41)

Hemel
Hempstead
Junction

A41 NEW KINGS LANGLEY BYPASS A41

St John's Road

BOXMOOR VILLAGE

Grand Union Canal

River Bulbourne

London Road

to AYLESBURY

(NOT TO SCALE)

*THE BOXMOOR
OSTEOPATHIC
PRACTICE*

9

Northridge
Way - No. 9

Moorland Road

Fishery
Road

British Rail
Hemel Hempstead

to BERKHAMSTED

To the memory of my Grandmother.

ACKNOWLEDGEMENTS

I would like to thank all the people who have made a contribution to this book. Many people have inspired me, by their questions, to include topics. Others, by their comment, have allowed me to continually develop and improve its content.

In particular I would like to thank Margaret Campbell and Roland Mann for their literary input and criticism.

A special thank you to my Mother for her suggestions and Frank Thompson for his photographic skill. I am also very grateful to Pat Moore-Searson for her encouragement.

CONTENTS

6. SELF HELP

7. TRAINING AND FITNESS

8. ARTHRITIS

9. PAIN AND STRAIN

1

ARE YOU SITTING COMFORTABLY?

My introduction to osteopathy came at a time when I had frequent back-ache. Like toothache, back-ache can be disabling. However, if you try to describe your pain to someone else you find that it is as difficult to explain as toothache is once the pain has gone.

That first visit to an osteopath made such a difference to my daily life that in my enthusiasm for this method of putting the body into good working order I decided I would like to have the skill to relieve others of their aches and pains.

Very soon after I set up my own practice, my patients' questions gave me to understand that they would like to have some hints on self help.

It is with this in mind that I have put together some ideas intended to prevent some problems, and some exercises to keep the body fit without strain.

2

ABOUT OSTEOPATHY

A VERY BRIEF HISTORY OF OSTEOPATHY

In 1874 Dr. Andrew Taylor Still started the first school of osteopathy at Kirksville, Missouri, U.S.A. From this small start osteopathy was brought to England in 1917 with the opening of the British School of Osteopathy in London.

WHAT IS AN OSTEOPATH?

An osteopath is a practitioner who works with his hands to relieve pain using a system of manipulation of the joints and soft tissues of the body. Some osteopaths also use machines which they feel will enhance the effects of their manipulation. Osteopaths do not all work in the same way. The treatment you receive will depend upon the condition being treated and its severity.

A Registered Osteopath will have satisfied the criteria required for acceptance onto the Register of Osteopaths. He or she will have a specified level of education and competence.

It is always advisable to go to a practitioner who has been recommended to you, either by your doctor or a friend. This way, when you see the osteopath you have a good idea of the type of treatment you will receive.

HOW IS AN OSTEOPATH TRAINED?

A Registered osteopath will have studied at a recognised College or School of osteopathy for a Diploma or Degree in osteopathy. Registered Osteopaths are recognised by the initials MRO (Member of the Register of Osteopaths) after their name.

I studied at The British School of Osteopathy (BSO) in London. The course at this college is full-time and covers a period of four years.

A thorough knowledge of anatomy (the study of the physical structure of the body) and physiology (the study of the way the body functions) is required by the osteopath. These subjects are studied at the BSO to about the same level as in a medical degree. Other areas studied include: embryology (the study of the structure and development of the body up to birth); neurology (the study of the anatomy and physiology of the nervous system); and other general medical subjects. Most important in the training of a Registered Osteopath is the time spent in clinical practice. In the four years' training provided by the BSO, over 1200 hours are spent in clinical training.

ARE ALL OSTEOPATHS THE SAME?

Some osteopaths are interested in sport related injuries, others specialise in the treatment of dancers.

For any hobby, sport, pastime or profession you may find an osteopath who spends much of his or her time treating these groups of people. This specialisation often reflects the particular interests of the individual osteopath.

Osteopaths may use techniques which vary considerably between practitioners. The style of treatment adopted will be that which the osteopath has found to be most useful and effective in their experience. They will then use techniques which are best suited to his or her size and strength.

CRANIAL OSTEOPATHY

A cranial osteopath uses subtle adjustments of the bones and connective tissues of the skull and sacrum (the base of the spine) to correct mechanical problems and relieve pain. Cranial osteopathy is often used to treat back and neck pain. It may also be useful when treating young children and babies as it is a very gentle form of manipulation.

Your local Registered Osteopath may be able to tell you if there is someone who practises cranial osteopathy in your area. He or she may also be able to tell you if this type of treatment is suitable for your condition.

VISCERAL OSTEOPATHY

Some osteopaths specialise in work on the internal organs, such as the stomach and the intestinal tract. These are practitioners of visceral osteopathy.

They apply subtle pressure to the abdomen, or related areas, to try to return a dysfunctional organ to its normal state. You may be told that avoiding certain foods or taking dietary supplements will help your problem.

Some of the conditions treated using these techniques are irritable bowel syndrome, and some menstrual problems.

OSTEOPATHY FOR CHILDREN

When a child is brought into an osteopath's surgery they have often undergone exhaustive medical tests in search of an answer to their problems. This invariably means that serious disease has probably been ruled out. The osteopath may often find that postural or mechanical problems are causing the trouble.

OSTEOPATHY FOR PREGNANT WOMEN

A regular spinal check-up may help to minimise back pain during your pregnancy. It may also help to prevent long term back trouble which can result from prolonged poor posture during your pregnancy.

Your osteopath will try to ensure that all of your spinal joints function as well as they are able while you are expecting your baby.

OSTEOPATHY FOR ANIMALS

Animals often respond well to osteopathic manipulation. The techniques used to treat animals will be modified to take account of the size and weight of the animal being treated. An osteopath who treats animals will normally work under the supervision of a veterinary surgeon.

CAN OSTEOPATHY HELP SOMEONE AT MY AGE?

Osteopaths are able to help patients of all ages, from young children to the very old. The osteopath has at his disposal techniques which allow him to help young children, where only gentle treatment may be appropriate. He also possesses the skills required to manipulate the biggest and toughest rugby player. Older patients may be treated using the gentle soft-tissue manipulation techniques appropriate to their age and physical condition. The osteopath will use techniques which he is certain are safe for the patient and which are both effective and as gentle as possible.

WHICH CONDITIONS ARE TREATED?

Some of the more common conditions which often respond well to treatment are backache, headache and any joint strain affecting the wrists, shoulders, hips, knees or ankles.

WHY SHOULD I CHOOSE OSTEOPATHY?

If you are in trouble with your back, neck or joints there are several therapies which you may look to for help. So why should you choose to visit an osteopath?

There are several good reasons. Firstly, osteopathy is a therapy which looks at the whole person and works with the natural healing system of the body. Secondly, osteopathy does not usually require you to take drugs and therefore does not have side-effects. Thirdly, an osteopath is a specialist in the treatment of spinal and joint injuries. The osteopath is able to recognise when a joint, muscle or connective tissue is causing problems and will treat these structures as and where appropriate. Fourthly, osteopathy is a one-to-one therapy, therefore you will be given the time and attention that your problem requires. Finally, and perhaps most importantly, the osteopath treats the cause of your problem not just your symptoms.

WHAT HAPPENS NEXT?

By examining your spinal joints and treating any problem areas the osteopath will try to ensure that every part of your spine operates as efficiently as possible. Having found out what is wrong with you and having decided that it may be possible to help you the osteopath will then begin a course of treatment. If each spinal joint does its fair share of the bending and twisting then the back usually compensates very well for any wear and tear.

MY FIRST VISIT TO THE OSTEOPATH

On your first visit to an osteopath you will be shown into the surgery and made as comfortable as possible. The osteopath will make a note of your personal details. Next you will be asked many questions about your problem to enable the osteopath to pinpoint the problem. If the osteopath considers that he can help you, you will be asked to undress down to your underwear. (Otherwise he will either refer you back to your doctor or suggest where you can get the help you need.)

The osteopath will examine you first in a standing position. You will be asked to move the injured area of your body through a full range of active movements. For example, if you are suffering with your low back you will be asked to bend (as far as you can without great discomfort) forwards, backwards, and from side to side, and to rotate your trunk from the waist to the left and right.

Don't be surprised if the osteopath examines your spine when you complain of pain in the arm or leg. An injury in one part of the body is often felt as pain in an apparently unrelated area. This type of pain is called "referred pain".

Now you may be asked to lie on a couch, or plinth. At this point the osteopath may carry out a series of orthopaedic and neurological tests. These are the same tests that doctors use when examining patients.

They help to guide the osteopath towards a particular diagnosis, or evaluation, of your problem.

In the case of a patient with a bad back or neck, the next stage of the examination may involve the osteopath checking your spinal joints by taking them through a range of movements.

This is done in order to determine whether they move freely, too much or not enough. If a joint in an arm or leg is in trouble the osteopath may take the affected joint through its full range of movements while the patient remains relaxed.

Finally the osteopath will palpate, or feel, the tissues using gentle manual pressure. He may at this stage be able to identify the muscle, joint or other structure responsible for your pain.

Once the osteopath has identified your problem he will decide on a course of treatment aimed at returning the injured structure's function to normal and eliminating, or reducing, your symptoms.

A consultation may include: useful advice, osteopathic joint manipulation, and exercises and treatments to be carried out at home. The number of treatments required, and the time between sessions, will be dictated by your particular problem and how quickly your body is able to respond to treatment and heal itself.

WHAT IS OSTEOPATHIC JOINT MANIPULATION?

One cause of back or neck pain is increased tightness, or tension, in the small muscles of the back or neck. The osteopath may choose to reduce this tension with the use of osteopathic manipulation.

This is not massage and may be explained by way of a simple example:

We may all have experienced how pain in a finger or toe joint can be relieved by pulling the offending joint until it clicks. The click is the result of a gapping, or separation, of the joint surfaces. The osteopath uses the same principle but in a far more sophisticated way, to treat disorders of the neck and back. It goes without saying that this sort of treatment should only be carried out by a fully trained practitioner.

There are many other types of manipulation used by osteopaths. Some of these are as follows:

Tight muscles respond well to kneading and stretching. This helps to increase the blood supply to an injured, or painful area and may help to speed the healing process.

A joint may be articulated by the osteopath i.e. moved through its pain-free range. Articulation helps to maintain movement in a damaged joint and will increase circulation to the area.

Friction, applied as a treatment to a damaged ligament, stimulates blood flow and may help to speed up the healing process. A ligament strain treated in this way often shows a spectacular improvement indeed you may be instantly symptom-free. However, this does not mean that you are fully fit, so please take note of any instructions you are given.

Give yourself at least two weeks away from hard physical activity even though you may be free of pain.

FOLLOWING MANIPULATION

Following manipulation, some form of exercise may be demonstrated or suggested. This will be given to you for a reason, it is advisable that you faithfully carry out any exercises you have been shown. To reduce inflammation regular treatment of the injured area with ice, or hot packs, may also be suggested.

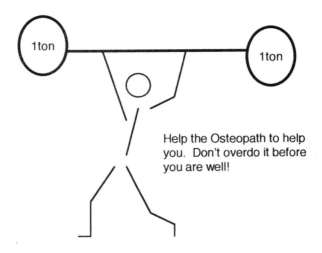

Help the Osteopath to help you. Don't overdo it before you are well!

WHEN AND HOW OFTEN SHOULD I SEE AN OSTEOPATH?

By periodically having your spinal joints checked, or "serviced" you may help to avoid the pain that can sometimes come about as a result of long-standing problems with some of the spinal joints.

It may be a good idea to look upon a visit to your osteopath as you would a check-up with your dentist. Regular maintenance treatment may help to prevent recurrence of a problem. A yearly "MoT" for your spine could help to keep your back in good order.

Generally speaking you will be asked to attend for treatment until you feel that your pain or symptoms have reduced to an acceptable level.

Not all problems can be sorted out in two or three treatments. In cases where a regular maintenance treatment is required, for example the treatment of a condition which is likely to recur, more regular attendance may be desirable.

Don't hesitate to discuss the likely timespan of your treatment.

AFTER TREATMENT

Occasionally a patient may feel sore following treatment. This is no cause for concern. The soreness should diminish or disappear over the next 24-48 hours. Cold treatment as described on page 33 may hasten the process.

Please do not hesitate to phone your osteopath for advice!

You will hopefully be in considerably less pain after treatment, and you may well feel stronger and more supple. This is no time for lifting heavy weights, jogging or catching up on the decorating. Your injury is still there and you must give it time to heal. That probably means two to three weeks of reduced workload and gentle exercises as prescribed by the osteopath. After this amount of time you may proceed cautiously with your normal day to day work.

3

DIET AND EATING

A SIMPLE GUIDE TO HEALTHY EATING

If you do not over-eat your weight should usually remain fairly constant. Many diets available today aim to achieve rapid weight loss. You may lose more weight in the long term if you control your food intake on a day-to-day basis. In this way you will neither starve yourself, nor over-indulge.

What follows is not a "diet", it is a series of tips designed to help you to get the most from the food you eat.

Always remove any excess fat from meat, which will not detract from the taste of the food but it will help you in your efforts to lose weight. Use the grill to cook meat which will help you to reduce your intake of fat. Eat fish once a week, grilled rather than fried.

Try drinking semi-skimmed milk which contains less fat.

Be sure to eat vegetables or salad every day. This will not only help to keep you healthy, but will provide a good source of vitamins and minerals.

You need fibre in your diet to keep your stomach and gut working efficiently. Eat fruit every day. There may be some truth in the old saying "an apple a day keeps the doctor away."

Try to make sure that at least two days per week are alcohol-free. Use these days to take your weekly exercise.

Only eat as much as you really need. Do not take second helpings especially if your job is sedentary.

Osteopaths are sometimes asked the question "should I be taking extra vitamins or supplements?" If you are already in good health and eat a sensible, varied diet you really should not need any extra vitamins or supplements if your diet is well balanced. Everything you need to thrive is present in the food you eat. Surplus vitamins are not stored in the body, so it is unnecessary to take extra with the idea that "if a little does you good, then more will be better."

Refined sugars should be avoided. If you eat a lot of this type of sugar it may lead to a series of highs and lows in your blood sugar levels throughout the day. This will make you feel full of energy one minute, then tired, then full of energy once more depending on when you had your last "fix" of sugar. If you must take snacks try a muesli bar (without added sugar), which releases energy slower than do sweets. This may help you to avoid highs and lows.

The amount of red meat and dairy products you eat should be kept to a sensible level. Sometimes people suffering with arthritis say that the pain they suffer is less if they cut down their consumption of these foods.

Keep your intake of tea and coffee down to just a few cups each day. Reducing your intake of these drinks may sometimes help to reduce anxiety.

If you suffer with migraine it may be worth trying to cut chocolate, cheese, strawberries and red wine out of your diet.

HOW OFTEN SHOULD I EAT?

Avoid eating between meals, eat three medium-sized meals per day. Have a cereal for breakfast with toast and fruit juice. Do not eat biscuits or chocolate mid-morning, but instead eat an apple or an orange. For lunch have a sandwich or a medium-sized meal. Remember that too much food at this time of day may make you drowsy and less effective at your work. Save plenty of room in your stomach for a cooked evening meal and always take a walk in the evening to help you to relax. Make this a part of your exercise routine.

It's no use starving yourself for three months in Spring to lose weight for your Summer holiday if you overeat all the rest of the year. What makes you put on weight is the total amount of food eaten each year not what you eat in one month.

4

AN INTRODUCTION TO THE BACK

WHAT IS THE SPINE AND HOW DOES IT WORK?

The spine is a jointed rod starting at the base of the skull and ending at the tailbone or coccyx. It supports the skull and body against gravity and protects the delicate system of nerves which run through the spinal canal (this is a channel which runs the length of the spine).

The spine is made up of individual bony building blocks. Each bone has a body (shaped like a small can of baked beans). Stuck onto the side of the body (the side of the can of beans) is a bony arch (rather like a hump-backed bridge). In the space between the body and the underside of the arch runs the spinal canal which contains the main nerves of the body (the spinal cord). On top of the arch (the bridge) is a bony point (imagine this as a man standing on top of the bridge) which is the bony bump which you can feel just beneath the skin of your back. There is one of these points on each bone in your back, some of which are more easy to feel than others. How easy they are to feel depends on how much muscle and fat you have in your body.

There are two more bony points, on each side of the one you are able to feel, which protrude from the sides of the arch of each vertebra. As these are covered with layers of muscle they cannot usually be located. Many of the muscles in your back are attached to these three bony projections. These structures act as levers and increase the pull that the spinal muscles are able to exert on each bone as they tighten or contract. The body of each bone, or vertebra, is the main supporting structure of the spine which holds the body upright against gravity. The arch with its bony projections gives the muscles in the back something solid to pull against as they contract.

There are a total of 33 bones, or vertebrae, in the spine. These are separated into 7 neck bones, or cervical vertebrae, 12 chest bones, or thoracic vertebrae. There are also 5 low back bones, or lumbar vertebrae and 5 sacral bones which are joined together into a solid wedge-shaped lump called the sacrum. Finally there is the tailbone or coccyx which is made up of 4 small bones fused together.

The neck bones are the most mobile in the spine. The topmost one is called the atlas, as it supports the skull; the second is the axis, which supports the atlas and skull. The atlas is able to pivot to the left and right on top of the axis. These top two bones are the most specialised ones in the neck. The other five are roughly similar in appearance. The neck can turn approximately 90 degrees to the left and 90 degrees to the right. The neck can also bend sideways, forwards and backwards.

THE HUMAN SPINE

The cervical spine (or neck) contains 7 bones. The topmost bone is called the atlas - it supports the skull. The bone beneath the atlas is called the axis - this bone allows the atlas and skull to rotate left and right. The atlas and the axis are the most specialised bones in the neck and there is no disc between them.

CERVICAL SPINE

The thoracic spine is made up of 12 bones. The ribs are attached in pairs one on either side of each bone or vertebra. The thoracic vertebrae together with the ribs form the rib-cage.

THORACIC SPINE

The lumbar spine (the low back) is made up of 5 bones.

LUMBAR SPINE

The sacrum is a block of 5 bones, it is wedge-shaped and the bones are fused together. The pelvis along with the sacrum forms a ring of bones which support the internal (abdominal) organs.

SACRUM

The coccyx is your tailbone, it is made up of 4 small bones fused together.

COCCYX

The 12 chest bones, or thoracic vertebrae are all fairly similar. These have the ribs attached to them. Together with the ribs they form a cage which houses and protects the heart and lungs. Because these vertebrae have ribs attached they make the chest area relatively inflexible but very strong.

The 5 low back bones, or lumbar vertebrae are larger in size than the others. They need to be strong to support the weight of the body. These bones move more freely than the chest or thoracic vertebrae but are not as mobile as those in the neck.

The sacrum is a group of 5 bones which are fused into one solid mass. It forms the keystone of the spine and its wedge shape helps to secure the spine in the pelvis.

The pelvis is a bowl-shaped bony ring, known as the hip bone, which helps to support the stomach, intestines and other internal organs. The pelvis acts as a stable platform helping to transfer power from the strong leg muscles to the rest of the body.

Attached to the end of the sacrum are another four bones which are fused together and called the coccyx. The coccyx has no function in locomotion in man. It is only ever noticed if it becomes damaged in a fall or following childbirth. If the coccyx becomes injured it can make sitting down a painful experience.

Now that we have seen how the spine is made it is important to understand how the bones are joined together.

If we can imagine the bones contained in the spine being piled one on top of another, we might assume that the resulting structure would be rigid and inflexible. In order to allow the spine to bend and twist, something flexible must be fixed between each pair of bones. Nature has provided just such a structure in the form of a cushion or disc. The discs are jelly-filled pads which absorb the shock of walking (rather like cushioned insoles in sports shoes). Each disc is stuck to the bottom of the bone above and the top of the bone below. The jelly in the disc is able to move around inside the disc but cannot escape from it. This movement of the jelly in the disc is what gives the back its flexibility, and allows one to bend forwards, backwards, sideways and twist to left or right. The disc with its jelly-centre works as shown in the following example: when one bends forwards to touch the toes the jelly in each disc is pushed backwards allowing more forward-bending. When one stands up again the jelly returns to its original position. Similarly, if you bend backwards the jelly will move forwards. The same principle may be applied to other movements as the jelly always moves in the opposite direction to the way the body is trying to bend.

One might imagine that if the discs in the back allowed a great deal of movement the body would be floppy and limp like a rag-doll. This is not the case because the small spinal joints which lie behind the disc on either side of the spine restrict spinal movement. The small spinal joints are found on the arch of the vertebra near to the side projections. Each joint articulates with the joint surface of the bone above it and the one below.

These joints, along with their ligaments (fibrous strengthening bands) and their joint capsules limit the range of movement of the back and stop one from moving too far in any given direction. The ligaments contain strong fibres which prevent excessive movement of a joint. The capsule of a joint is like a bag which surrounds the joint, protects it, and limits its range of movement.

Because the small spinal joints limit the range of movement at each level in the spine the different areas of the spine have been forced to specialise. Some parts are better at moving in one direction than another. If you suffer with pain in the back or neck it is important to understand this as certain movements will tend to upset the mechanics of the spine leading to painful consequences. The movements of the spine are briefly discussed below.

The small spinal joints in the neck lie roughly horizontally allowing the neck to rotate and bend forwards and backwards easily. However, because of this setup the neck is not very good at bending sideways.

In the chest area the small spinal joints are angled so that it is easy to bend forwards and backwards, but rotation in this part of the spine is restricted. This area is also stiffened by the ribs.

In the lumbar spine (the low back) the small spinal joints will allow you to bend forwards and backwards easily, however, bending left and right are more restricted.

Between each pair of bones there are nerves which protrude from the spine, one from each side. These nerves exit the spinal column by passing between the back of the disc and the front of the small spinal joint. This leaves a small aperture through which each nerve passes. This is usually large enough to allow for the passage of the nerves; but sometimes, if there is damage to a disc or one of the small spinal joints, one of these nerves may become slightly squashed leading to pain in the arm or leg.

WHY DOES THE SPINE GO WRONG?

If the ingenious system of a flexible disc sandwiched between two bones eventually breaks down it will lead to back-pain and disability with which some of us suffer. The jelly inside each disc is always looking for a way to escape as it is under quite considerable pressure. As we get older the outer edges of the disc may become frayed or damaged, which may be caused by a fall or a traffic accident. In older people even if there has been no obvious injury, the discs tend to contain less jelly. This "drying-out" of the discs can lead to a loss in height with age, and the back becomes less flexible.

Damage to the outside of a disc can sometimes lead to seepage of the jelly from the disc due to the pressure. Once the jelly has started to leak it cannot be replaced and the disc may be somewhat flatter than it was before (a bit like a rubber ball with too little air in it). Leakages from the disc are called herniations.

These leakages may press on pain sensitive structures, such as ligaments and cause aches and pains. If a disc bulge presses on a nerve the resulting pain may be felt in your arm or leg. This type of pain may be severe and is sometimes accompanied by weakness in a limb or by pins and needles (tingling) or numbness in the skin which is supplied by the nerve. Until this pressure from the bulging disc has reduced, the pain tends to continue. Sometimes if the nerve is badly damaged the pain may last for a long time even though the pressure on the nerve has been reduced (nerves take a long time to heal once they have been damaged). However, in most cases pain will only last for a week or two.

THE INTER-VERTEBRAL DISC

Jelly centre of the spinal disc (or nucleus pulposus). This can move about inside the disc.

Strong fibrous cartilage. Holds jelly contents inside the disc.

Vertebral body. The bony building block of the spine. The disc is sandwiched between two of these.

A DISC HERNIATION

(A disc and a vertebra seen from above)

Leaking jelly from disc. Once it has leaked this jelly will not return to the disc.

The jelly centre of the disc may leak if the fibrous disc breaks down. If the jelly presses on a nerve it will cause pain and may damage the nerve.

5

GENERAL HEALTH

SMOKING

Nowadays even the most seasoned smoker must be aware that smoking is hazardous and causes serious diseases. If you smoke you have an increased chance of dying before you retire. Smokers may be wasting not only their pension contributions but also their lives!

Your osteopath will be able to suggest ideas that may help you in your attempt to give up smoking. One idea is to replace cigarettes with some form of exercise. You might find that the "buzz" or "high" you feel after an exercise session may help to reduce the desire for a cigarette. Exercise won't leave you with bad breath or smoky clothes either!

Breathing other peoples' cigarette smoke, known as passive smoking, is now recognised as a serious health risk. Therefore you should avoid working in smoke-filled rooms and never smoke when there are young children in the room. Passive smoking may damage the delicate tissues in a young child's chest and lungs.

If you have already given up smoking it should be reassuring to note that you may already have increased your life expectancy.

OSTEOPATHY IN PREGNANCY

During pregnancy the increased weight you are carrying will affect the mechanics of your spine, which will suffer if it is put under too much stress or made to work too hard. The result may be the onset of low back pain or other aches and pains of mechanical origin.

These symptoms may be reduced or eliminated by the use of gentle osteopathic manipulation while you lie on your side. You should of course tell your doctor about any treatment that you are taking, as well as any symptoms you experience in the course of your pregnancy.

ARE YOU AN OPTIMIST?

How you come to terms with illness may have some bearing on the speed at which you recover from it. Certainly, people do appear to cope differently even when suffering from the same illness.

A good example of one person's response to pain is the following: the sufferer thinks "My back is still causing me a lot of pain every day. I see no end to this terrible experience!" This is a sad-and-sorry way to look at illness.

It might be better to be an optimist and think "Now my back is causing me pain for less of my day than it used to. This is real progress, there really is light at the end of the tunnel!" The level of pain experienced by both patients was the same, only the attitude of the sufferers was different.

It is very natural to feel down at heart when you are in pain. Try to build up the positive side of your illness and see it as an opportunity to develop other talents. Take up drawing or painting. You may find that you are another Picasso!

6

SELF HELP

SOME USEFUL ITEMS

Several items that you can buy without prescription at the chemists can be a helpful supplement to osteopathic treatment.

They include:

- Anti-inflammatory drugs such as Nurofen. (Be sure to tell the pharmacist if you are taking other medication on prescription!)

- Special ice packs and heat packs. These are costlier but no more effective than the home-made substitute: a bag of frozen peas wrapped in a towel for the cold pack, a hot-water bottle for the heat treatment.

- Freeze and heat sprays. These are a great convenience for patients who have to go to work, but they are less effective than real ice packs and heat packs.

COLD TREATMENT

One of the best methods of self-help, when carried out under the osteopath's guidance, is to regularly ice the site of injury (provided the skin is unbroken) with a bag of frozen peas wrapped in a thin towel. Ideally this should be done for ten minutes every waking hour for 36 hours, or as close to that as your daily routine permits.

HOT AND COLD TREATMENT

Following a course of cold treatment, alternate cold and hot compresses will further promote healing. As before, a bag of peas wrapped in a thin towel will serve as your cold pack, while a hot-water bottle similarly wrapped will provide the heat.

First, you apply the cold pack for just five minutes; then the hot-pack, for another five minutes; then cold again, hot again, and finishing with cold -- 25 minutes in all. This ideally should be repeated every hour until the pain is relieved. If you can't manage 25 minutes every hour, reduce the length of the alternate cold and hot applications. As little as two minutes each of the cold-hot-cold-hot-cold sequence -- 10 minutes in the hour -- will be of benefit. Whatever the length of treatment, always start and finish with cold.

THE RULE OF RICE

In general an injury is best treated in a standard way. This is a set of rules, called the rule of **RICE** and is set out below:

Rest - Rest is often of benefit to a new injury. This should be a period with relatively light duties. It may also include specific exercises which are carried out on a regular basis and are designed to speed the healing process. Your osteopath will tell you which exercises may suit your problem.

Ice - Place an ice pack wrapped in a thin towel on the affected area - 10 minutes per hour.

Compression - A bandage will support a new injury - Not good in the long term.

Elevation - If there is swelling hold injured area above heart height to aid drainage of fluid.

If there is severe swelling or bruising then go to casualty pretty quickly.

Always go to casualty with head injuries.

7

TRAINING AND FITNESS

DAILY FITNESS

Many of the injuries the osteopath sees are the result of over-enthusiastic indulgence in some sport or other strenuous activity by people who are basically just not very fit. Regular exercise is the surest way to improve general health and avoid the so irritating and painful injuries that often accompany enthusiasm.

Habitual postures, like sitting at a desk or leaning over a sink or work bench, may may tend to shorten some muscles (like the hamstrings), and cause others (like the postural muscles in the back) to become tense. By regularly taking your joints through the whole of their normal range of movement you can reduce the strain on your body -- and, for that matter your mind.

What follows is a gentle five minutes-a-day programme that you can use to get your body toned up. You may decide to exercise your legs on day 1, your back on day 2, and your shoulders on day 3. The cycle will then begin again, and you will have the basis for a varied non-boring exercise routine.

Begin slowly and build up over a period of weeks and months. Not only will you feel fitter in body but your self image may improve, that, in turn, will show in the way you relate to others.

If you are pregnant do not embark on an exercise programme before consulting your osteopath or your doctor.

EXERCISES

The following exercises are intended for improving flexibility and general muscle tone.

They may also be used to warm-up before playing sport or taking part in fitness training.

LEG ROUTINE:

1) Stand one pace away from the back of a high chair. Keeping your back straight, clasp the chair-back with both hands.
Stretch right leg forward and swing to right and left in front of body 10 times.
Repeat exercise with left leg 10 times.

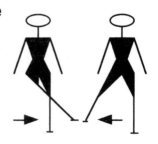

2) Stand with right side to chair-back. Clasp the chair-back with right hand.
Swing right leg forwards and backwards 10 times.

Reverse sides and repeat exercise.

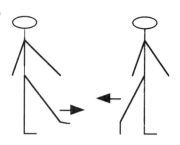

3) Stand with right side to back of chair. Clasp chair-back with right hand. Stretch right leg one pace backwards keeping foot flat on floor.
With back straight, bend left knee as far as possible. Hold position for 10 seconds.
Reverse sides and repeat.

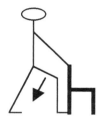

4) Stand facing chair-back. Legs stretched comfortably apart. Clasp chair-back with both hands. Bend each knee in turn as far as possible without discomfort.

Hold position for 10 seconds each side.

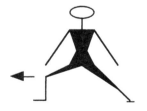

5) Stand facing chair-back. Hold chair-back with right hand. Bending left knee, raise left foot backwards. Clasp left foot with left hand and pull upwards.
Hold position for 10 seconds.

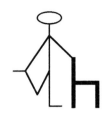

Reverse sides and repeat.

6) Standing one pace from back of chair. Put right leg one pace forward. Keeping the back straight and both feet flat on the floor, bend the right knee to feel the left calf stretching.
Hold for 10 seconds.
Reverse sides and repeat.

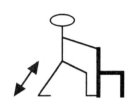

7) Hamstring stretch: Stand facing chair-back. Put the left leg back one step. Keep your hips square to the chair-back. Bend the right knee to 45 degrees. Keeping the back straight, lean forward towards the chair until you feel the stretch in the back of the right leg. Hold for 10 seconds.
Reverse sides and repeat

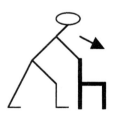

BACK AND ABDOMINAL EXERCISES:

8) Lie on back.
Clasp hands round knees. Whilst breathing out pull knees towards chest (to a count of 4 seconds).
Relax slowly whilst breathing in (to a count of 4 seconds).

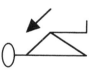

Repeat 10 times.

9) Lie with back on the floor, legs in the air, knees bent with calves and feet resting on the seat of the chair. Lift head slowly off the floor and then gently lower again.

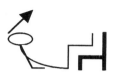

Repeat slowly 10 times.

10) Lie with back on the floor, legs in the air, knees bent with calves and feet resting on the seat of a chair. Raise head and shoulders slowly off the ground. Gently turn your torso to the left and then to the right. Return to the central position. Lower to floor.
Repeat slowly 10 times.

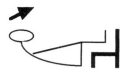

11) Stand up, stretch your left arm towards the ceiling, lean sideways as far as is comfortable to the right.
Repeat this exercise 5 times.

Reverse sides and repeat exercise.

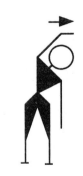

12) Stand upright. Raise your arms sideways level with your shoulders. Keep your hips straight. Gently twist torso to left and right.
(Do NOT bounce to get extra movement).

Repeat exercise 10 times.

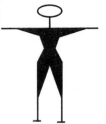

UPPER BODY/SHOULDER EXERCISES:

Carry out the following exercises slowly and in full. Do not force any movement; use your breathing to increase your range of movement. To increase the amount of movement, breathe in before you carry out a stretch and breathe out as you stretch.

13) Shoulder circles: Stand upright. Raise your arms sideways level with your shoulders. Slowly make small circles in a forward direction with your arms. Gradually increase size of circles and then decrease them again. Do this exercise for 10 seconds and then repeat, this time rotating your arms backwards.

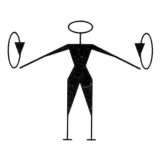

14) With your right hand clasp your left elbow and pull it as far as possible to the right across your chest. Hold this position for five seconds.

Reverse sides and repeat exercise.

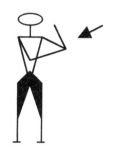

15) Raise your arms above your head. With your right hand clasp your left elbow and pull it as far as possible to the right over your head. Hold this position for 5 seconds.

Reverse sides and repeat.

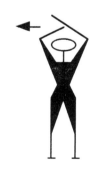

16) With both arms behind your back, clasp your left wrist with your right hand and pull as far as possible to the right.

Reverse sides and repeat the exercise.

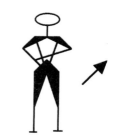

17) Shrug shoulders and make circles...

...forwards 10 times.

...backwards 10 times.

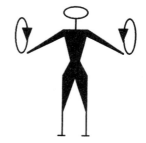

18) Sit upright on chair. Stretch to full height. Allow neck and head to drop gently forward. Roll head from left to right.
Repeat this exercise 5 times.

(Never stretch backwards or look at ceiling to relieve pain)

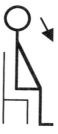

side view

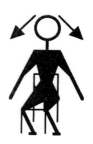

front view

SPECIAL EXERCISE SECTION

These exercises are used to treat specific conditions and are therefore listed separately.

Abdominal breathing exercises are used to reduce muscle tension. They are particularly useful for relieving stress. This type of exercise must be practised every day and the technique should then be carried into everyday life as an effective method of relieving tension.

Pendular arm swinging and the knee strengthening exercise are important exercises and should be used when you are recovering from any shoulder or knee injury.

19) Abdominal breathing exercise:
On a comfortable surface lie on your back with a pillow under your head. Place one hand on your chest. Place the other hand on your abdomen. Relax your arms and shoulders keeping your hands in place. Breathe deeply and slowly.
Ensure that the hand on your abdomen rises and falls with the breath. Continue for 4 minutes.

In these exercises the hand on the chest neither rises nor falls.

Advanced exercise:
1) Breathe in to a count of 4.
2) Breathe out to a count of 6.
3) Hold breath to a count of 4.
Repeat from 1 and continue
for 6 minutes.

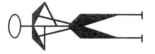

20)   Pendular arm swinging:
Stand facing the back of a chair.   Lean the trunk of the body forward to about 30 degrees.   Grasp back of chair with one hand. Allow the other arm to hang freely in front of you. Gently swing your arm in small circles (no more than 12 inches in diameter).
After 30 seconds repeat in reverse direction

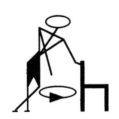

21) Knee strengthening exercise:
Sit on a chair with your legs together.

Tense the muscles on the front of your thighs by straightening your legs. Hold this contraction for 4 seconds.

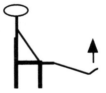

Relax and repeat 10 times.

Do this at least twice a day.

IMPORTANT NOTE:

IF PAIN IS EXPERIENCED ON ANY EXERCISE
STOP IMMEDIATELY!

WHO SHOULD EXERCISE?

Everybody should exercise, however the amount of exercise you do will depend on your age and your general health. If you are under 35 years old it is fairly safe to carry out most of the currently available exercise programmes. If you have any doubts about your health then it is safer to consult a doctor or your osteopath before you begin to train. If you are over 35 years old, and are not used to exercising, please be sensible and get advice from a doctor or your osteopath on the best way to start to train.

WHY SHOULD YOU BE FIT?

You don't have to be fit to live to a ripe old age. But common sense will tell you that there are benefits to be gained by maintaining your body in good condition. You will be able to carry out hard physical tasks for longer periods, and you will increase the strength and efficiency of your heart.

Exercise, along with a sensible diet, will reduce the amount of fat that you carry. You won't necessarily lose weight because exercising builds muscle, and muscle is heavier than fat. Conceivably, you could even gain weight through exercise, though this is unlikely. What is certain is that you will improve the shape and contour of your limbs and body and tone up your abdominal muscles. As a result you will look both slimmer and healthier.

The increase in abdominal muscle tone you gain by exercising will act as a muscular "corset", which will strengthen your back helping to protect you from injury. This is why the exercise routines in this book emphasise abdominal muscle strengthening.

MAKE FITNESS A PART OF LIVING

Whilst you should not become obsessive about fitness, it is a good idea to develop the habit of exercise so as to make fitness a part of living. The "stop-start" type of fitness training is far less healthy than a steady programme that follows you through life.

Perhaps the most effective and safest exercise is regular, brisk walking. Get used to walking to the shops rather than driving, especially if the distance is less than half a mile or so.

While you work you can be exercising. For instance, if you are sitting on a chair sit upright, grasp the sides of the seat and try to move your arms out to the side, then use the same resistance to try to pull your arms in towards your body. This type of exercise is excellent for toning muscles and making you aware of your posture. By using your imagination you could make your office or desk into your own personal fitness centre.

SLEEP AND FITNESS

Sleep is a necessity of life. Without enough sleep you will very quickly become run down and lose physical conditioning and mental alertness. What is important in sleep is more the quality of rest, than the amount, which varies from person to person.

A simple exercise routine or a brisk walk in the fresh air before retiring will help to relax and calm you.

A small snack and a warm drink (not tea or coffee) will help you to get off to sleep. Do not go to bed hungry.

Make sure your bedroom is as dark as possible, quiet, and that you are warm but not too hot.

It is most important to try to leave your worries and troubles behind when you go to bed. Try to keep your mind on pleasant things or happy memories, in order to distract you from brooding or worrying.

If you follow these principles and learn and practice a relaxation technique, such as abdominal breathing, you will soon be fast asleep.

STRENGTH AND FITNESS

So far we have been concerned with increasing and maintaining flexibility of the joints. At this point we can look further into increasing strength and cardiovascular fitness.

Along with the increase in flexibility you may already have achieved through following the flexibility exercise routine you may now wish to increase the workload you can achieve using a strengthening routine. This build up of power will be realised over a longer time period than the increase in flexibility you have already achieved and you should proceed with care so as not to hurt yourself.

To increase your strength you must stress your joints and muscles using repetitive exercise carried out three times per week. This period of exercise will last for forty minutes **(you may begin with twenty minutes until you are fitter)** and is preceded by ten minutes warming up using the flexibility exercises numbers 1-18. Following the forty minute routine you will spend another ten minutes warming down, using the same routine you used to warm up.

Please remember that if you have a preexisting medical condition, are pregnant or are taking any long term medication, you would be well advised to seek medical advice before embarking on a vigorous exercise programme.

WHAT IF I BECOME INJURED?

If you suffer an injury, for whatever reason, turn it into a learning experience. Learn how to avoid similar problems in the future by avoiding certain movements or exercises. Turn each weakness into a strength and never give in to negative thinking. This principle may be applied to sporting injury or to life experiences in general.

Positive thinking will help you to overcome obstacles that may seem insurmountable at the time.

REST AND FITNESS

If you remember that an essential part of any fitness programme is rest, you will progress faster and achieve more in the long term. It is in the period of rest between training periods that your body is building itself up in readiness for the next workout. If rest is insufficient, or if you overtrain, your body will become overtired and you will be heading for injury.

ILLNESS

Never train while you are ill. If a period of illness interferes with your training rest up until you feel totally well again. Use the time to gently improve your flexibility by carrying out one or two stretching exercises per day. This will help the time pass more quickly and give you a sense of achievement.

Remember: To exercise when you are unwell is counterproductive as well as potentially dangerous.

HOW HARD SHOULD I WORK?

Do not work through pain. Pain is your body's way of saying "slow down and rest." Take note of what your body is telling you. If you follow this rule you will become stronger more rapidly and avoid injury.

HOW AND WHY SHOULD I CHECK MY WORK RATE?

It is important for anyone taking part in a fitness programme to avoid overworking. The safety aspect of training cannot be overemphasised. The end result of overtraining is usually injury. To avoid hurting yourself and to protect your heart it is a good policy to restrict your exercise to not more than 70% of the maximum of which you are capable. Your heart rate is a good indicator of how hard you are working. The faster it beats the more work you are doing. Your heart rate may be measured quickly and easily while you are exercising. The way this is done is set out below:

Find the pulse in one of your wrists, it is found about 2 inches from the base of your thumb on the palm side of your forearm. Use gentle pressure from your index finger to feel the pulse. Count the beats for 15 seconds and multiply by four to get the number of heart beats per minute (or heart rate). Your resting heart rate is best taken first thing in the morning before the stress and strain of daily life begins. Before you exercise your resting heart rate will probably be somewhere in the region of 72 beats per minute, if you are in good health.

Take your pulse once a day for seven days, add the daily readings and divide the sum by 7 to get the daily average. Now that you know your normal resting heart rate, you can use it to decide whether to exercise or rest.

If at any given time your resting heart rate is not significantly higher than normal you may carry out an exercise session. Otherwise you will be well advised to rest until your heart rate is normal once more.

While exercising take your pulse three times. Try to keep your heart rate above 90 beats per minute but no higher than 135 beats per minute, unless you are under expert supervision. If your heart rate rises above 135, or if you feel unwell **STOP AT ONCE.**

RECOVERING FROM EXERCISE

After exercise, check your heart rate at three-minute intervals for 9 minutes. As you get fitter, your heart rate will fall more quickly back to its normal resting speed. Keep a record of your heart rate after exercise. If you find that it is taking longer than usual to slow down, you may be overtraining. You should increase your rest time and reduce training time accordingly.

WHAT IS CARDIOVASCULAR EXERCISE?

This exercise is aimed at strengthening the most important muscle in your body, your heart. You will help to maintain your heart and blood vessels in good condition by exercising regularly. The amount of this type of exercise you will carry out very much depends on your age and physical condition.

If you have any doubts about your heart, or general health, consult your doctor before exercising vigorously. Especially if you are over thirty five years of age. Whichever form of exercise you choose, build up slowly starting with five or six minutes training increasing over the weeks to the full exercise time. Stop when you feel you have had enough. Do not expect to achieve the same level of performance every time you train.

BREATHING AND EXERCISE

When you train your breathing should always be steady and controlled. If you are getting out of breath you are probably overworking and you should slow down until you are once more breathing at a steady rate. When you carry out any exercise a general rule is that you will breathe before contraction of a muscle and breathe out with the effort of contracting it.

HOW MUCH WEIGHT SHOULD I USE WHEN I TRAIN?

If you use weights to train it is important, if you are to avoid injury, that you understand how heavy the weight you use should be. **Never use any weight that feels heavy at the start of an exercise.** A weight should be easy to hold and not cause any pain anywhere in your body.

To save money start off by using everyday household objects as weights. Two cans of baked beans make an excellent alternative to a set of hand weights.

When you carry out an exercise you are loading your muscles and joints to make them work, thus making the muscles stronger. If a load feels heavy at the start of an exercise routine it will certainly be too heavy for you by the time you finish, and may well cause injury. **If in doubt, do not do it!**

SO TO WORK

Provided you are feeling well and are suffering no medical condition that makes exercise inadvisable, you should now go through the DAILY FITNESS exercise routine. Work through slowly and deliberately from exercise number 1 to number 18. Carrying out the exercises slowly in full will take approximately ten minutes. Check your heart rate now. If you are at the lower end of the range in which you want to work, you are ready to begin with one of the cardiovascular exercises.

The following exercise routine is harder than it might at first appear so please take your time and do not overwork your body.

CARDIOVASCULAR EXERCISES

Carry out exercise (1) or (2) but not both at each session. Do not allow your heart rate to increase above 135 beats per minute in this or any other exercise.

Cardio-vascular exercise (1)
Take a brisk 20-minute walk.
Start slowly and gradually build up your speed, slowing down for the last 5 minutes. Check your pulse twice to be sure you are exercising within your upper and lower limits.

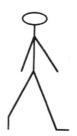

Cardio-vascular exercise (2)

Stand at the bottom of a flight of stairs. Hold banister with one hand. Step up to first step with one foot, then bring the other up to join it. Step down with first foot, then bring the other one to join it. Repeat for 3 minutes.

Change sides. Starting with second foot repeat exercise, continue for 3 minutes, then change sides again.

Continue for 12 minutes alternating every 3 minutes **(check your pulse twice in the exercise period).** Work only as long as you can without getting out of breath or feeling ill. As you become fitter you will work for 18 minutes.

If your pulse does not rise, hold a small weight in each hand for extra workload or step up using two steps instead of one.

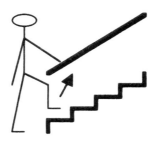

GENERAL EXERCISES

1) Sit ups:
Lie with your back on the floor, knees bent at right angles, feet flat on the floor. Place your hands next to your ears, but do not hold your head or ears. Raising your head and shoulders off the ground, bring your head towards your knees, breathing out as you come up.
Turn your torso to the left and then to the right. **Return to the central position**. Lower to the floor breathing in as you come down.

Repeat 15 times. As you get stronger increase this to 30 times.

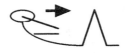

2) Extension:
Lie on your front, arms along your sides. Breathe in. Lift your head and shoulders off the floor whilst breathing out to a count of 4 seconds.
Relax slowly whilst breathing in again to a count of 4 seconds.

Repeat 10 times.

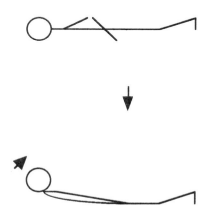

3) Shoulder circles:
Hold a small weight or a dumbbell in each hand. Shrug shoulders and make circles...

...forwards 10 times.

...backwards 10 times.

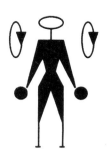

4) Forward raise:
Stand with your feet eighteen inches apart, one foot in front of the other. Hold a small weight or a light dumbbell in each hand.
Breathe in.
With the weights in front of you and your elbows slightly bent, breathe out slowly and raise the weights to shoulder height (**but no higher than this**) in front of you.
Slowly lower the weights as you breathe in.

Repeat 10 times.

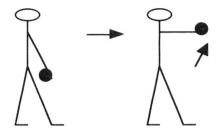

5) Lateral raise:
Stand with feet 18 inches apart.
Hold a light weight or a
dumbbell in each hand. **Bend
elbows** (45 degrees is
enough) and breathe in.
As you breathe out raise the
weights sideways up to shoulder
height (but no higher).
Lower your arms slowly to sides
as you breathe in.

Repeat 10 times.

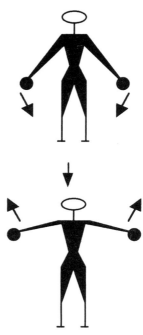

6) Triceps strengthening:
Put one foot 2 feet in front of the other. Keeping your back straight, lean forward to 30 degrees. With your elbows bent to 90 degrees, hold a weight alongside your hips. Breathe in.
As you let your breath out, straighten your arms backwards. **Maintain a straight back at all times.**
Breathe in again as you bend your arms to the start position.

Repeat 10 times.

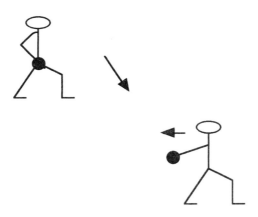

7) Bicep curl:

Stand with your arms at your sides, a weight or small dumbbell in each hand.

Breathe in.

As you breathe out, flex your elbows to bring the weight to shoulder height.

Slowly let the weights down to your side as you breathe in again.

Repeat 10 times.

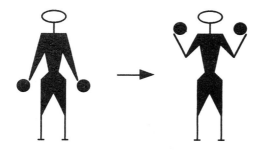

8) Press ups:

These are an excellent all round exercise. They use your chest muscles, abdominal and leg muscles. Adopt a position lying on your front with your hands, palms down, at your sides at the level of your shoulders.

Breathe in deeply, breathe out and push your body away from the floor keeping as straight as possible, slowly but strongly, until your arms are locked straight.

Lower your body, slowly under full control, to the floor as you breathe in.

Repeat 20 times, or as many times as you can without causing pain in your back or arms. **See half press up if this is too difficult for you.**

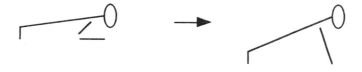

9) Half press up:
People with less upper-body strength may find it easier to do a press up leaving the knees on the ground.

Adopt the same starting position as for the full press up. Start to breathe out as you slowly push your body away from the floor, allow your knees to remain in contact with the ground while you push up.

Concentrate on keeping your back straight and as flat as possible. When you have locked your arms out straight start to come slowly to the floor again as you breathe in, bending your elbows as you come down.

Repeat 10 times. Increasing to 20 times as you get stronger.

10) Overhead press:
Stand with your feet 18 inches apart. Hold a weight
or small dumbbell at shoulder height with your arms
at your sides.
Breathe in.
As you breathe out push the weight above your
shoulders until your arms are straight and above
your head at shoulder width. Slowly bring the
weights back to shoulder height bending your arms
and breathing in as you do this.

Repeat 10 times.

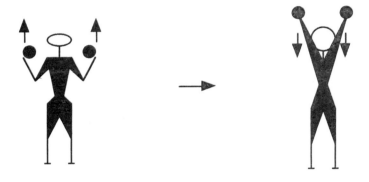

11) Calf raise:

Stand on a step holding the banister. Only your toes and the balls of your feet should rest on the edge of the step.

Breathe in.

Breathe out as you push your body upwards using only your toes and the balls of your feet. Allow your body weight to stretch your calf muscles as you lower your body (at the same time breathing in).

Repeat 20 times.

To make this exercise harder, use only one foot to push you up, tucking the other foot behind the ankle you are working.

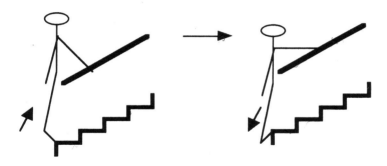

12) The squat:
Stand facing a high backed chair 18 inches away. Hold the chair back with both hands. Keeping your back straight and as near to vertical as possible, breathe in as you bend your knees to 90 degrees or as near to this as you can (do not squat to more than 90 degrees). Slowly return to the starting position.

Repeat 20 times.

To make the exercise harder hold a weight in each hand and do not hold the table. A book placed under each heel will help you maintain your balance.

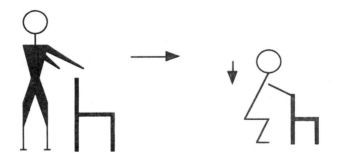

13) Side bending waist exercise:
Stand with your feet 18 inches apart. Hold a small
dumbbell or weight in one hand at the side of
your body. Stand as tall as you can. Lean to the
side holding the weight. Take the arm holding the
weight down the side of your leg, breathing in as you
lean to the side (not forward or back). When you
have leant over as far as is comfortable, come
back to the starting position slowly, breathing out
as you come up.

Repeat 10 times.

Change hands and exercise the other side of your
waist.

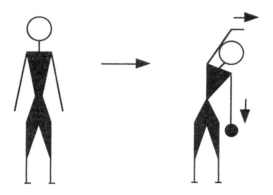

14) Lie on your side on the floor. Support yourself with your arms in front to ensure that you are in a stable position. Take a deep breath, breathe out slowly and raise your upper leg sideways towards the ceiling. Do not allow your trunk or hips to twist out of line. Lower your leg slowly as you breathe in.

Repeat 10 times.

Change sides and repeat.

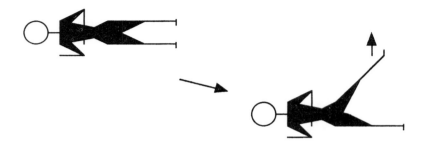

15) Lie on your back with your arms by your sides, legs flat on the floor, feet together. Lift one leg off the floor up to 90 degrees or as high as you can, (breathing out as you do so). Keep both legs straight as you exercise. Lower the raised leg slowly, breathing in as the leg is brought down.

Repeat 5 times each side.

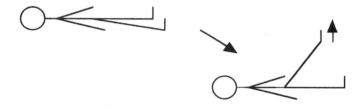

16) Leg extension:
Lie on your front, arms along your sides. Breathe in.
Lift one leg up 6 inches (but no higher) off the floor
whilst breathing out to a count of 4 seconds.
Relax slowly whilst breathing in, again to a count of
4 seconds.

Repeat 5 times each side.

If you suffer with pain in your low back take care with this exercise and lift your leg only one inch from the floor.

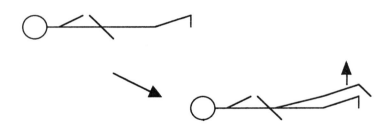

8

ARTHRITIS

WHAT IS ARTHRITIS?

Arthritis is perhaps one of the most emotive words in the dictionary, bringing to mind deformed joints, pain and disability. Sadly, this image is valid in some cases, but in the great majority the condition is far less aggressive.

The word arthritis means inflammation of a joint. In many cases the inflammation can be reduced with treatment, and pain will diminish along with it .

Among the many different types of arthritis, one of the more common encountered by osteopaths is osteoarthritis.

OSTEOARTHRITIS OR "WEAR AND TEAR" ARTHRITIS

This form of arthritis often begins in the 30s and increases inevitably with age. Osteoarthritis may be brought on by repeated trauma to the joints, but often factors such as obesity, occupation and postural problems increase the likelihood of its developing. The condition is especially common in the spinal, knee and hip joints.

Patients complain of stiffness and aches and pains, especially when the joint has been immobile for some time. Where the spine is arthritic, nerves supplying the limbs may be affected, leading to pain in arms and legs.

Osteopathic treatment of osteoarthritis will be aimed at keeping the joint mobile and maintaining the strength of muscles which control the joint and reducing or controlling pain. The osteopath will also advise the patient on how to protect his or her joints from further damage or injury.

Osteopaths are often asked the question "I have been told that I have osteoarthritis can I reduce the pain I am suffering by altering my diet?" There is no guarantee that a change in your diet will lessen the pain you suffer. However, many people feel relief when they cut down their intake of certain foods. Some of those which, if they are eliminated from the diet, may give relief from pain are:

Foods containing gluten such as bread and cakes. Gluten is a protein present in cereal grains (especially wheat) so avoid any food containing wheat-flour.

Citrus fruits such as oranges and lemons should be avoided. These fruits contain citric acid. Resist the temptation to buy foods which contain this chemical as a flavouring.

Tea and coffee may be cut out of the diet. Dandelion coffee may be used instead of these drinks if refreshment is needed.

9

PAIN AND STRAIN

WHAT IS PAIN TO ME?

Pain is a very difficult thing to describe, it is different for every individual and what may be unbearable to one person may be quite acceptable to another. If you are in pain and others do not seem to understand or accept that you are suffering this can be very frustrating.

Pain can be felt constantly or intermittently, it may be sharp or dull, aching, searing or feel like a knife twisting between your ribs. The words used to describe pain are countless and locating the pain or its source may be even more difficult, especially if the pain is only present for some of the time.

Ask questions until you are clear in your mind that you understand your problem. Long words may be confusing and even frightening, yet they are often simply descriptions which health professionals use to describe common conditions in order that they can be understood by their colleagues. If you understand the origin of your pain or problem you may find that the fear and anxiety you feel will reduce and therefore the pain will diminish.

WHAT IS REFERRED PAIN?

Sometimes, when you see an osteopath or doctor, you may be told that the pain you are suffering with is coming from a part of your body which is some distance from the part that hurts. For instance: a patient presents at the osteopath's surgery with pain running down the back of one leg into the foot. The osteopath having examined the patient tells him that he has injured a disc in his low back. To many people this might sound faintly ridiculous until they are shown a model of a human spine and it is pointed out that the nerves coming out of the spinal canal run close to the vertebral discs. These nerves may be interfered with by a damaged spinal disc. This may result in pressure on the nerve which can lead to pain, tingling, numbness or weakness in a part of the leg corresponding to the nerve which is in trouble.

This type of pain, felt at some distance from its source is called **referred pain.**

In the same way that pain is sometimes felt in the leg when the problem, or injury, is in the low back it is possible to feel pain from neck injury in the arm, shoulder or hands. The cause of these pains is often the result of pressure on the nerves as they leave the spine in the neck.

LEG LENGTH DIFFERENCES

Many patients are amazed if they are told that one of their legs is longer than the other. They would be less surprised if a shoe shop measured both feet and found that they had a half-size difference in foot length. We have come to accept a difference in the size of our feet.

In both cases the cause of the length difference is the same. During growth one limb stops lengthening before the other. In a four legged animal this difference would usually go unnoticed. However, as we stand on only two legs the resulting tilt of the pelvis can, after many years of life, lead to a breakdown of the body's compensation mechanisms. In some cases this may lead to pain in the low back or elsewhere. Many people go through life with a slight difference in leg length with no problems.

Sometimes a patient may gain considerable relief from their pain with the use of a small lift in the heel of one shoe. This would usually be worn in the shoe of the shorter leg.

LOW BACK PAIN

There are many structures and organs in the body that can cause pain in the low back. If other, less straight forward, causes of pain in the low back have been eliminated it is possible that a mechanical problem is to blame for the pain.

Muscles, ligaments and joints are just a few of the pain sensitive structures which can lead to pain in the low back.

Today many people live a sedentary lifestyle. This is especially noticeable when compared with previous generations. This relative inactivity can lead to weakness of the back muscles which are then liable to become damaged, along with other structures in the spine. We are most at risk when we become more physically active in holidays and at weekends. The modern trend towards DIY has led to many days away from work with strained backs. Similarly heavy lifting at work among employees who are less than totally fit can lead to time off work.

Osteopaths successfully treat many millions of people suffering with low back pain each year. Patients may be treated using techniques developed to stretch the soft tissue structures in the low back.

You may also be treated using osteopathic manipulation, this is used to correct mechanical problems in the small spinal joints.

NECK PAIN

Due to the relatively large range of movement found in some of the neck joints it is common to find injuries in this area. Taken along with the injuries caused by "whiplash" accidents this makes patients with neck problems a common sight at the osteopath's surgery.

Treatment of these injuries is similar in principle to that of low back problems, only the techniques are modified to take account of the smaller size of the neck as compared with the lumbar spine.

THORACIC OR MID-BACK PAIN

Pain in this region of the back is common and is often the result of poor sitting or standing posture. The spine in this region is stiffened by the ribs, this reduces the likelihood of some problems but presents other hazards. Straining the small rib joints can be extremely painful, especially when it comes to breathing. This type of injury usually responds well to osteopathic treatment which often may involve manipulation of the affected joint.

Avoiding recurrence of mid-back pain involves analysing sitting and standing posture, and advice on correct lifting and bending techniques.

SHOULD I WEAR A CORSET OR NECK COLLAR IF I AM IN PAIN WITH MY BACK OR NECK?

The question "Should I wear a soft collar, support belt, or corset?" comes up time and again. There is no easy answer. There are two sides to the argument:

Firstly, if you wear a support of any kind for any length of time the muscles which give strength to a joint may become weaker, or lazy.

Secondly, if a joint is inflamed there may well be a need for support, this will be required until the inflammation has subsided.

Important Note: Every injury, or problem, is different. If you are in a lot of pain then it may be necessary to give extra support when driving or doing manual work.

Never forget: Pain is the body's way of saying "slow down or rest" so be sensible and listen to what your body is telling you.

TENNIS ELBOW

Stand upright, your arms by your sides with the palms of your hands facing the front. Look at your elbow, the side of your elbow furthest from your body has a bony feel to it.

In tennis elbow this bony point, where the muscles which bend your wrist backwards join to form a tendon, becomes very tender and painful. The cause of this is not only a poor backhand shot in tennis, but also overusing the arm in a screwdriving type of movement.

The condition is often successfully treated osteopathically by reducing the tension in the wrist muscles, resting the arm, and reducing inflammation applying ice packs to the painful point. If the original injury action is avoided the problem will often not recur.

GOLFER'S ELBOW

If you find the opposite side of your elbow to the one found to locate a tennis elbow injury, you will feel that there is a similar bony point on the inside of your elbow. In golfer's elbow, sometimes caused by overuse of the wrist in golf, there is pain around this bony point.

As in tennis elbow treatment is aimed at restoring the forearm muscles to their normal tone. Along with ice packs applied regularly, rest and exercises, the condition often resolves quickly.

FROZEN SHOULDER

In a true frozen shoulder there is pain experienced at night, movements of the shoulder are restricted and the condition may last for eighteen months. This may seem disheartening, however, some conditions of the shoulder may be wrongly labelled as frozen shoulder but with treatment recover very quickly, so it is best not to lose heart.

With vigorous exercises encouragement and manipulation of the joint healing may be speeded up.

KNEE PAIN

Within and around the knee joint are many structures capable of causing pain and swelling, clicking noises and locking of the joint.

It is important to get knee problems treated as the muscles which protect the joint will become weak very quickly. This weakening of the muscles is storing up trouble for later on in life. As soon as an injury occurs, **after seeking advice on your condition**, the strong knee muscles should be worked using a knee strengthening exercise.

You should not continue with sport or running until the pain has gone.

THE SPRAINED ANKLE

The ankle joint is very easily twisted or turned inwards resulting in pain inflammation and swelling of the joint. The outer side of the joint is likely to be damaged because this part of the joint is more mobile than the inside. This allows the ankle to roll inwards and results in tearing or straining of the ankle ligaments. In a straight forward ankle strain rest is recommended along with ice packs regularly applied to the ankle. An ankle support, or bandage will help to control the swelling.

The ankle should be rested in a "feet-up" position, using a foot stool while watching the television is a good idea.

If the ankle does not respond to this treatment or bruising is present it is a good idea to seek medical advice.

THE ARTHRITIC HIP

The hip joint is a very resilient joint, it can, and does, put up with a lot of abuse. When the hip does eventually start to cause problems it can be very disabling, and painful. When a hip is shown to be wearing, for example as a result of an X-ray investigation, do not give up hope.

Painful or worn hip joints often respond very well to treatment using manipulation of the joint and work on the soft tissues that surround the joint.

A gentle exercise routine, carried out along with regular stretching of the hip and lower limb muscles, will often reduce symptoms to an acceptable level. This will help to preserve the range of movement of the affected joint.

Regular **light use** of an exercise bicycle may be of considerable help with this type of problem. **Do not overdo the exercise**, listen to your body and if it starts to complain rest up for a few days.

HEADACHE

Headache is a common problem complained of by many patients. There are many causes of headache, most are fairly simple and will clear up by eating meals at regular intervals, taking adequate rests as you work or getting enough sleep at night. If headaches are a regular feature of your day, or are getting progressively worse, medical advice should be sought.

If you suffer with tension headaches it is a good idea to analyse your sitting posture. Do you constantly slouch and create tension in your neck? This can lead to headache, as can sitting too long in one position at work. Get up and walk around for a few minutes every hour, this simple remedy may help to reduce the tension in your back and neck muscles.

If you spend a lot of time on your feet make sure that you keep your weight equally spread on both legs, try to stand back on your heels, and stand tall at all times.

SHINGLES

Herpes zoster, or shingles, is a virus infection which attacks a nerve and the area of skin supplied by the nerve. It is caused by the reactivation of a virus which is present in the patient's body. The patient at some time will have had chicken pox but there is no evidence that shingles may be contracted from someone suffering from chicken pox or shingles. One or more nerves on the same side of the body may be affected.

Shingles may occur at any age, but it is rare in childhood and is most often seen in patients over the age of fifty.

Pain is usually the first symptom this will run from the start of the nerve affected to the skin supplied by the same nerve. The skin may be very painful in this region.

Three or four days after the pain starts a rash will appear which consists of closely grouped raised nodes (swellings). These then develop into small blisters the tops of which are filled with clear fluid, they are found in groups often around one side of the trunk. The skin in the affected area is a reddish colour. A few days later redness subsides and the blisters dry into crusts leaving small scars. The skin in the affected area may become partly or completely numb. Pain may last for weeks, months or longer.

Recognising shingles is not possible until the rash appears, once it is seen you should consult your doctor.

STRESS

Stress is a necessary part of living. Without some pressure to get on with things nothing would ever get done. The time when stress becomes a problem is when the good stress, needed to succeed in life, becomes bad stress which a person is unable to deal with. Many factors will govern your response to stress, support from family members will often help you come to terms with problems.

If you are unable to gain support from a friend or a relative stress counsellors are becoming more readily available and The Samaritans have a branch in most areas.

YOGA

Yoga is a form of exercise that will improve your flexibility and teach you how to relax. By increasing flexibility you will help protect your joints from injury. The benefits of learning to relax are that you will feel more at ease with yourself and with others.

Not everybody will take to this form of exercise, but unless you try it you may never realise what you are missing. If you do start with a class give yourself at least a couple of months regular attendance before deciding whether you like it or not.

REHABILITATION FOLLOWING A STROKE

Many people who have had a stroke are left with some degree of disability. The speed of recovery from a stroke depends on the amount of damage to the nervous system and "The will to live," or motivation, of the patient.

Following a stroke nerve and brain tissues are damaged, the muscles supplied by injured nerves may become smaller and wasted. These wasted muscles may give rise to aches and pains, because they are not being used as they were before the stroke.

Many patients gain much relief from these problems with help from osteopaths who may treat them (if and where appropriate) using osteopathic soft-tissue manipulation techniques.

10

SPORT

AVOIDING INJURY IN SPORT

With the increase in leisure time available, which has come about due to reduced working hours, there has been a trend in recent years towards sport as a recreation and a means of improving general health and fitness. As a direct result of this increase in sporting activity there has been a rise in sport related injury. Many of these injuries are avoidable. There are two ways to enjoy sport, the first is "fast and furious" where the newly recruited athlete tries to emulate his favourite sporting superstars. This athlete may soon come unstuck and very quickly end his new sporting career at the injury clinic, never to participate again for fear of reliving the pain of injury. The other alternative is the "slow and steady" school of thought.

"Slow and steady" is the safest introduction to any sport.

Even if you were a great sporting person in earlier years do not assume that you are immune to the rigours of time.

A steady programme of stretching and a gradual introduction to sport is always to be recommended.

When you are warming up for sport try to visualise each part of a game and the individual components which go to make a good shot or set piece.

Visualisation will prepare your mind and body for the vigorous exercise which is to come.

Like all great campaigns the game is planned well before it begins. Planning will include buying well fitting sports shoes. These will avoid damaging your joints due to the substantial shock which is transmitted all the way from your feet to the base of your skull, when you accelerate from a standstill or try to slow down rapidly.

Spend at least ten minutes warming up and a similar time following the game warming down.

The approach which often leads to excellence is rarely aggressive, always controlled, planned in advance and practised regularly both mentally and physically.

Injury will be less likely and you will recover from injury much more quickly if your fitness plan builds strength slowly and you practise your skills regularly.

CANOEING

Canoeing in calm water may be useful for building upper body strength. Shoulder strength will increase as a result of the powerful paddling action required to propel a canoe through the water. Equipment should include a modern life jacket and safety helmet.

Shoulder injuries may respond well to this exercise, as may mid-back problems. If your trouble is in the low back you should take care to learn correct lifting techniques. Trouble will start when you attempt to lift a canoe filled with water.

Most sports centres will have a club where safe canoeing may be learned and practised before going out in open water.

For safety's sake go canoeing in groups and leave white water and sea canoeing to the experts.

CYCLING

Cycling is a good exercise for strengthening your legs, improving stamina and is good for the heart and lungs. As with any exercise, if you are a beginner, take it easy when you first start. If you begin with a short ride then you should avoid stiffness in your legs the next day.

If you get problems with your neck a bicycle which allows you to sit upright, such as a mountain bike, will help you to avoid neck pain. Bicycles with dropped handlebars, the old style racing bike, force your neck to arch backwards and can sometimes lead to neck trouble, especially if you are already a sufferer.

FOOTBALL - RUGBY - HOCKEY

If you play rugby, football or hockey it is likely that you have a team coach, or trainer. This is the person who, when you would rather get on with the game, insists that you spend time stretching out, and warming up, your arms, back and legs. Without this preparation there would be far more injuries on the pitch.

It might pay you to spend a few minutes of each day stretching your muscles. The length of your sporting career depends on you staying fit and avoiding unnecessary injury. Many people wait until they are nearing the end of their sporting life to start taking the warm up, and stretching, seriously.

It would be more sensible to start stretching while you are young and make your career in sport last longer! Spend a few minutes each day carrying out DAILY FITNESS exercises 1-18.

You may find that your flexibility improves by a surprising amount. This discipline will help to keep you in sport, and injury free. Try it!

GOLF

Golf is an excellent way to get fit. It combines walking several miles in the fresh air with the powerful driving action necessary to move the ball long distances down the fairway, and intense concentration and fine movement control when you reach the green.

In order to avoid straining your low back, often the result of poor technique or over enthusiastic driving, you should complete a full stretching routine as a warm up, and a similar routine after the game.

This also applies to work on the driving range. Exercises in DAILY FITNESS 3-18 will prepare you and help to prevent avoidable injury.

HORSE RIDING

This sport is very good when it comes to strengthening the leg muscles, however there is an in-built hazard in horse riding, that is there is a tendency to fall off, among some riders. The results can be painful, as anyone who has fallen will agree.

A good 10 minutes warm up using DAILY FITNESS exercises 1-18 will prepare you for your sport, and a warm down following a ride will help to prevent aches and pains.

RACQUET SPORTS

Games such as tennis, squash and badminton are, generally speaking, one handed sports. A possible result of playing this type of sport is that injury may arise in the playing arm. For example, a right handed tennis player is more likely to develop a right than a left sided tennis elbow. This, and other injuries, may be the result of poor technique, or overuse of the racquet arm.

One way to improve poor technique is to take lessons with a good, qualified, sports coach.

Once an injury has occurred remedial treatment should begin at once. To continue to play with an injury can only prolong the agony. Neglecting an injury may also make it a longer job to treat, and therefore it may be more expensive, when you do eventually seek assistance.

With all racquet sports a full 10 minute warm up before the game (you may use exercises 1 - 18 in the DAILY FITNESS section) and a similar period of warming down following the game is essential. Attention to flexibility will help to avoid unnecessary injury and time away from your sport.

RUNNING

Of all the different types of exercise running is perhaps the one which is most likely to cause you problems. Some of the more obvious injuries caused by running are sprained ankles and twisted knees. If you have had problems with your back then running is a good way to start the troubles off again.

Having said all this running or jogging burns up a lot of energy very rapidly and can help with weight loss if carried out in moderation.

If you wish to take up running you should start getting fit by going for brisk walks. If you are over 35 years of age you should check with your doctor whether you are fit enough to run.

When you start to run begin with a half mile course, aim to complete this and still be able to talk without being out of breath. Train at most three times per week. When the half mile run is becoming too easy try to run for one mile.

Do not attempt at this stage to time the runs, just aim to finish them comfortably. As you improve you may increase the distance you run and in time your speed will increase naturally without conscious effort.

If it is your intention to run in half or full marathons you would be wise to join an athletic club as the companionship will help you to train. The many experienced runners in a club will help you avoid too many mistakes and injuries.

SWIMMING FOR FITNESS

Swimming is an exercise which will improve your overall level of fitness whilst avoiding potentially damaging impact to the joints which so often accompanies other active sports. There are, however, some problems which accompany certain strokes in swimming.

Breaststroke will often aggravate neck problems because it forces you to arch your neck backwards. If you have had trouble with your neck in the past you would be wise to avoid this stroke in favour of backstroke or front crawl.

If you intend to go swimming it is as well to stick to a regular time in order that you establish a habit because you will gain most from swimming if you go regularly. Twenty minutes swimming three times a week is enough for general fitness.

Swimming lengths can be tedious so try to use different strokes and swim one length fast and the next slow, this will give added interest.

SWIMMING TO RECOVER FROM INJURY

Just as swimming is an excellent form of fitness training it can also be used when you are recovering from an injury. Shoulder, knee, ankle and back injuries often respond well to this type of non weight bearing exercise.

You should begin slowly and build up over a period of weeks starting with just 10 minutes in the pool splashing around. Swimming three times per week will be enough for most people.

If you train in a large pool start with just three or four lengths per session and increase this number by one or two lengths each week. Build up to fifteen or twenty lengths per session after several months.

WEIGHT TRAINING

Weight training can be used as an aid to recovering from an injury, or it can be included in a whole body fitness plan.

When used in recovery from illness or injury the aim of training is to first identify a weakness, in a joint or body part, and then to target this for specific strength building exercises. When used as a sport, weight training is useful for building confidence or to prepare the body to take part in games where more than average strength is needed.

WEIGHT TRAINING TO RECOVER FROM INJURY

Following a period of immobilisation, of a joint, there will be wasting of muscle with weakening of the affected joint. In order to return the joint to normal, in as short a time as possible, a routine of stretching the affected area, using flexibility exercises, is undertaken.

Under instruction or supervision, a series of exercises, targeting the muscles controlling the injured area, is carried out. The type of exercise will depend on the area to be worked. The intensity of training is matched to the severity of the injury, this will be decided by the therapist assessing and treating the injury.

WEIGHT TRAINING AS A SPORT

When carried out in moderation, and on a regular basis, weight training can be an effective part of a fitness plan.

The most important part of training is the warm up and the warm down. These should each be of at least ten minutes duration. Each should aim to stretch out all joints and muscles which are to be exercised in any training session. This will help to prevent injury and make arrival at the required fitness level much faster.

Training sessions should be of at least forty minutes duration (20 minutes of this time is the recovery period between exercises). At first train twice a week, this will rise to three times per week after several months training.

For a beginner it is a good idea to train at a sports centre where a basic training is given before you are allowed out on your own. The training machines vary widely, all have some benefits and some disadvantages, these will be evened out if a good balanced training schedule is used.

Free weights may be used to train, however these can be dangerous especially when using very heavy weights.

The training session should include at least ten minutes cardiovascular exercise, an example of this is the use of an exercise bicycle.

Whatever the reason for training with weights, any exercise should be carried out in full control and the weight used should not be so heavy that you are unable to complete the exercise you intend to carry out.

11

POSTURE

POSTURE IN CHILDHOOD

Poor postural habits picked up in childhood may lead to back and neck pain in later life. If postural adjustment Is carried out early in life it is possible that the effects of some injuries might be minimised.

It is unusual for children to suffer with back pain.

If they are in pain it should be investigated. If medical investigations prove that there is nothing sinister causing the problem then it is possible that a postural problem may be to blame.

Children copy the way their parents and friends stand, sit and walk. It is therefore possible that faulty postural habits may develop as a result of copying the behaviour of others. This may lead to aches and pains at an age when you do not normally expect them. As an example, if a parent has an unusual way of walking then you may find that a young child, doing what comes naturally to children, copies the parent and the result may be a young person with painful heels, knees or low back pain.

It may not be noticed by parents that their child has taken to constantly slouching or stamping around the room. An outsider may be the first to notice, or the child may start to complain of headache or backache. Sometimes unusual wear and tear on the soles of the shoes may be the first sign of a problem.

What can be done to prevent these problems?

Firstly, it is not a good idea to become paranoid about the way a child sits or walks. Everybody slouches for some part of the day, problems only arise when it becomes a constant habit to walk stooped and sit hunched up like a question mark. A few well chosen words of advice may be all that is needed to avoid problems. Alternatively some form of training such as ballet or gymnastics may give a person a better idea of a more ideal posture.

Generally, the earlier a problem is tackled the easier it is to solve.

SITTING POSTURE

Much of your day is probably spent sitting down in a chair. If you slouch, with an unsupported lumbar spine, for much of this time you may well be straining your back unnecessarily. It is a good idea to sit well back in your chair, if the seat is very soft place a cushion behind you to prevent you from slumping into the seat. You should also avoid chairs which put a lot of pressure onto the backs of the thighs.

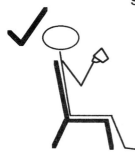

If you spend time sitting and relaxing try not to slouch in your chair. Use a chair with an upright back and place a cushion behind your back for extra support - especially if you suffer with your low back!

STANDING POSTURE

When you take into account all the different ways that it is possible to stand it becomes clear that to describe the perfect posture is pretty well impossible. There are, however, times in the day when you may be able to adopt a more ideal standing posture. When you are waiting in a queue or simply standing still you may be able to influence the way in which you hold yourself.

First consider your feet. You may find that by wearing a more comfortable pair of shoes, or a pair of cushioned insoles, you are able to reduce tiredness. If you stand still for any length of time you will reduce tension in the backs of your legs if you try to stand back on your heels, rather than on your toes.

Keep your knees straight and the feet 12 to 18 inches apart. Feel the pressure from the floor on the bottoms of your feet, this should be equal so that you are evenly balanced and the weight taken on each foot is the same.

Now hold in your tummy, by tensing your abdominal muscles, the effect of this is to flatten your low back and reduce back ache.

Finally, try to imagine a piece of string pulling up from the top of your head, stretch your neck upwards by tucking in your chin. This will reduce neck tension and pressure on the small joints in your neck.

Here you have a posture that will help you to lessen fatigue and reduce aches and pains if practised regularly.

12

EVERYDAY ACTIVITY

USING AND HOLDING THE TELEPHONE

A very common way to upset the mechanics of the neck is to habitually hold a telephone between a raised shoulder and the ear. This will lead to increased tension in the muscles of the neck and can cause stiff necks and headaches. If your job involves using the telephone for much of the day you might find one of the headsets available on the market useful. This will allow you to keep your head in a more normal position while you work.

When using the telephone always make a conscious effort to sit upright, hold the handset in one hand, and avoid raising your shoulders, no matter how heated the discussion.

GARDENING THE PAIN FREE WAY

1. Put off till tomorrow half of what you planned to do today. Gardening is heavy work, being too keen to finish a project can prove costly in pain and time off work with injury. Moderation in all gardening activities will allow you to enjoy the garden all summer long.

2. Watering plants is often essential to ensure a good crop or a beautiful display of flowers. However, lifting a heavy watering can above your head to soak hanging baskets is a neck injury waiting to happen. Always fill the can with just enough water for each basket, or use a milk bottle and refill it from a tap or bucket. Never carry a watering can if it feels too heavy, you can be sure it will be even heavier by the time you reach your destination. Half empty the can then try again (remembering to conserve water).

3. Digging the garden is the last straw for many a long suffering back. Trouble may come if you use a spade that is too heavy, or attempt to finish a long job in one go. Spend no more than ten minutes at a time digging. Leave the job and go off and pot up a few bulbs or tomato plants. You may return to the digging now, or better still do a bit each day. Never work if you are in pain - It can only get worse. Try and keep your back upright and straight. Bend from your knees to avoid straining your back when you dig. Keep the blade of the spade in front of you at all times, do not bend your back and twist from the waist at the same time.

PAIN FREE GARDENING

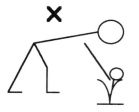

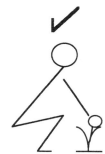

Know the weight of an object before you lift it. Especially if it is anchored to the ground!

Use your knees when you need to bend. Keep your back straight. DON'T BEND FROM THE WAIST!

4. Sweeping grass clippings or leaves: too much bending and twisting will play havoc with your back. Always keep your back straight, allow your legs and arms to do most of the work. Avoid sweeping large piles of rubbish or grass which may be too heavy for you.

5. Always know the weight of an object BEFORE you lift it. When you do lift something keep your back straight and vertical, now bend from the knees get a good grip and lift. Before lifting anything know where you are going to put it down.

CUTTING THE GRASS

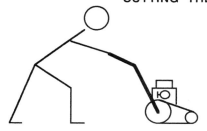

Take care when pull starting your petrol mower. Use your arm strength not your back. If the mower will not start get it serviced - don't get angry with it!

SAFER PAINTING AND DECORATING

Painting and decorating is one of those forms of exercise which you take up on moving house or just whenever the spirit moves you. This is often late at night after work, or when the children are asleep. If this is the case then it is likely that you will be tired and therefore more likely to be injured.

Most common among decorating injuries is the sore neck which may be caused by painting high walls or ceilings. This involves holding a brush or roller above shoulder height for prolonged periods of time, arching your neck backwards, and straining either the neck or the shoulder doing most work. A very simple way to reduce your chances of neck or shoulder strain would be to buy a broom handle or an extending roller handle from a hardware shop. Fix the roller to the end of this handle and this will allow you to roll the wall from the floor without stretching your neck backwards.

When you work with a roller on a pole always keep your arms below shoulder height. Another common way to injure yourself while decorating is to fall off a chair or stool. If you must use one then make sure that the stool or chair has four legs, all of which are in contact with the ground, this will give you a good stable platform.

If you use a chair with a back make sure that the back is either in front of you or to the side, this will prevent you from toppling over if you accidentally step back or lose your   balance.

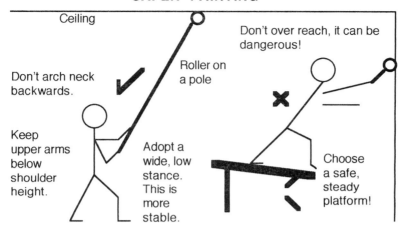

If you are unsteady on your feet, ask a competent friend to paint any difficult to reach places. Always consider using a professional to paint or hang paper in a stair well, it is very easy to fall when working in this part of the house.

HOW DO YOU SLEEP WITH A BAD BACK

You may find that getting off to sleep is very difficult while you are suffering with your back. There are a few things which you may find helpful. A pillow placed under your knees as you lie on your back will often relieve the pain sufficiently to allow you to sleep. If this is not enough then using an ice pack for ten minutes will often do the trick. Finally, if all else fails, you may need to take an anti inflammatory drug, such as Nurofen.

SLEEPING WITH A BAD BACK

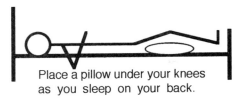

Place a pillow under your knees
as you sleep on your back.

Never lie on your front when you are in pain with your back, this will only aggravate your condition. Find the most comfortable position and try to relax yourself by reading a book or listening to the radio until sleep overtakes you.

CAR DRIVERS

Driving a car is best avoided if you are suffering with a bad back. However, if you are obliged to drive then it is important to bear in mind a few things. If you spend too long in one position your back will become stiff and painful. To stop this happening make sure that you have adequate support for your back. Placing a cushion in the small of your back will prevent you from slumping and avoid more discomfort later.

SAFER CAR DRIVING

Don't allow your shoulders to rise up around
your ears, even in the longest traffic jams.

Ensure adequate
low back support
in your car. Use a
small pillow as a
lumbar roll.

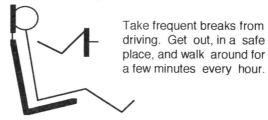

Take frequent breaks from
driving. Get out, in a safe
place, and walk around for
a few minutes every hour.

Make sure your car seat does not press
into the back of your thighs as you drive.

Move your seat every ten minutes. You probably
have at least two controls on your car seat. One
controls the distance from the control pedals, another
controls the angle of the seat-back. Move the seat
position a little at a time, first forwards, then
backwards a few minutes later.

Now, make the seat more upright, later make it
recline a little. For safety's sake the car should be
stationary when these adjustments are made. In this
way you will prevent your back from becoming "set"
in one position and thus enable you to drive longer
without discomfort.

Make frequent stops, at least one every hour. Walk
around for a few minutes. The time lost by taking
breaks will be very little and you will arrive at your
destination safer, fresher and in much less discomfort
than would otherwise have been the case.

Carry a can of a freeze spray with you on your journey, this will make a good first aid kit for a sore back. Always consider the alternative, that is to ask someone else to drive.

VDU OPERATORS AND DESK WORKERS

Unless operators of VDU's and desk-bound workers adopt good posture at their work, it is likely that headache and backache will become a regular occurrence. Whilst it may be tempting to slump into your chair the long term effects of poor posture will soon start to show. It is easy to avoid problems if you spend a little time thinking how you might adjust your work environment to suit your body.

WORKSTATION SETUP

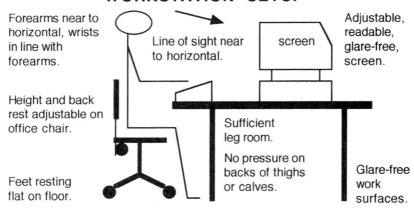

Forearms near to horizontal, wrists in line with forearms.

Line of sight near to horizontal.

screen

Adjustable, readable, glare-free, screen.

Height and back rest adjustable on office chair.

Sufficient leg room.

Feet resting flat on floor.

No pressure on backs of thighs or calves.

Glare-free work surfaces.

Seat height should allow your feet to lie flat on the floor without the feeling that the edge of your seat is pressing into the backs of your thighs. Sit well back in your chair and ensure that the back of the seat holds the curve of your low back firmly.

If you do not have an adjustable seat, place a small cushion between your low back and the back of the chair in order that you do not slouch.

If you have a well adjusted sitting posture it will make it difficult to slouch and you will avoid straining your back.

Desk height should allow you, when sitting, to gently rest your forearms on the desktop without leaning forwards and upsetting your posture.

If you use a VDU the screen should be positioned so that it is at, or near, eye level. The keyboard is set up so that your elbows are close to your sides and the forearms are at right angles to the upper arm. In this position your fingers will rest gently on the keyboard with your wrists in line with the forearms.

You should stand and walk around at least once every half hour to avoid back and neck pain.

13

GENERAL INFORMATION

USEFUL ADDRESSES AND TELEPHONE NUMBERS

AA help-line for people with disabilities to provide advice and information on aspects of mobility for disabled motorists: Free calls on (0800)262050. People owning Minicom should dial (0800) 887766 which alerts staff that a hearing problem driver needs help.

Al Anon Family Groups
61 Dover Street, London SE1 4YF.
tel.: 071 403 0888

Alcohol concern
305 Grays Inn Road, London WC1X 8QF.
tel.: 071 833 3471

Alcoholics Anonymous
11 Redcliffe Gardens, London SW10 9BG.
tel.: 071 352 3001

ARMS (Action and Research for Multiple Sclerosis)
4a Chapel Hill
Stanstead
Essex
CM24 8AG
tel.: 0279 815553

Arthritis Care
18 Stephenson Way
London NW1 2HD
tel.: 071 916 1500

Ash (Action on Smoking and Health)
102 Gloucester Place, London W1H 3DA.
tel.: 071 637 9843

Association for Post-Natal Illness
c/o Claire Delpech
7 Gowan Avenue
London SW6 6RH
tel.: 071 731 4867

British Tinnitus Association
Room 6. 14-18 West Bar Green
Sheffield S1 2DA

Carer's National Association
29 Chilworth Mews
London W2 3RG
tel.: 071 724 7776

Chest Heart and Stroke Association
Tavistock House
North Tavistock Square
London WC1H 9JE

Counsel and Care for the Elderly
Lower Ground Floor, Twyman House,
16 Bonny Street, London NW1 9PG. Provides a free comprehensive
advisory and information service to elderly people and their carers on
issues such as accommodation, benefits and respite care.

CRUSE - Bereavement Care
Cruse House, 126 Sheen Road, Richmond,
Surrey TW9 1UR.
tel.: 081 940 4818

Dark Horse Venture
Unit D54, South Brunswick Dock, Liverpool L3 4BD
Aims to discover the hidden talents of older people, through new
activities.

Depressives Anonymous
36 Chestnut Avenue, Beverley,
Humberside HU17 9QU.
tel.: 0482 860619

Disabled Drivers' Association
Ashwellthorpe Hall
Ashwellthorpe
Norfolk
NR16 1EX
tel.: 0508 41449
(10am-3pm plus answerphone)

Disabled Living Foundation
380-384 Harrow Road
London W9
tel.: 081 289 6111

Extend (for Advice on exercise for the elderly)
1A North Street, Sherringham, Norfolk NR26 8LJ.
tel.: 0263 822479.

Hyperactive Children's Support Group
71 Whyke Lane
Chichester
West Sussex
PO19 2LD

Lupus Group Arthritis Care
5 Grosvenor Crescent London
SW1X 7ER
tel.: 071 235 0902

Manic-Depressive Fellowship
51 Sheen Road
Richmond
Surrey
tel.: 081 940 6235

Mind (The National Association for Mental Health)
22 Harley Street, London W1N 2ED.
tel.: 071 637 0741.

Narcotics Anonymous
PO Box 246, c/o 47 Milman Street, London SW10.
tel.: 071 351 6794/6066.

National Ankylosing Spondylitis Society
5 Grosvenor Crescent
London
SW1X 7ER
tel.: 071 235 9585

National Back Pain Association
31-33 Park Road
Teddington
Middlesex
TW11 OAB
tel.: 081 977 5474

National Childbirth Trust
Alexandra House, Oldham Terrace, London W3 6NH.
tel.: 071 992 8637

National Osteoporosis Society
PO Box 10, Radstock
Bath
Avon
BA3 3YB
tel.: 0761 32472

National Waiting List Helpline
Help for patients seeking a shorter waiting list
in other districts
tel.: 081 558 1551

Patients' rights association, 18 Victoria Park Sq, London E2 9PF
tel.: 081 981 5676

Psoriasis Association
7 Milton Street
Northampton
NN2 7JG
tel.: 0604 711129

QUIT: Smokers' quit line. tel.: 071 487 3000.

Radar
(Royal Association for Disability and Rehabilitation)
25 Mortimer Street
London
W1N 8AB
tel.: 071 637 5400

SCODA: (Standing Conference on Drug Abuse)
1-4 Hatton Place, Hatton Garden, London EC1N 8ND.
tel.: 071 430 2341/2.

Scoliosis Association (UK)
380-384 Harrow Road, London W9 2HU.
tel.: 071 289 5652
Aims: To promote awareness about the condition which results in
curvature of the spine in order to ensure early diagnosis and treatment.
Also offers advice to sufferers.

Society of Teachers of the Alexander Technique
10 London House
66 Fulham Road
London SW10 9EL

Technical Equipment for Disabled People
Hazeldene
Ightham
Sevenoaks Road
Kent
TN15 9AD
tel.: 0732 883818

The British Paraplegic Sports Society (BPSS) has changed its name to
The British Wheelchair Sports Foundation.   There is also a new logo
incorporating the brand name "wheelpower".   Guttmann Sports Centre,
Harvey Road, Stoke Mandeville, Bucks, HP21 9PP.

The Centre for Pregnancy Nutrition has opened Eating in Pregnancy and
Pre-pregnancy help-line on 2nd September at the University Department
of Obstetrics and Gynaecology, Northern General Hospital, Sheffield.
Staff will man the help-line on weekdays between 10am and 2pm.   At all
other times there will be an answering service, which aims to respond
within 24 hours.   tel.: 0742 424084.

The General Council and Register of Osteopaths, Ltd,
56 London Street, Reading, Berkshire, RG1 4SQ.
tel.: 0734 576585

The Global Project in support of the United Nations Decade of Disabled
Persons is at Room 109, 11 Belgrave Road, London SW1V 1RB.
tel.: 071 834 0477.   Fax: 071 821 9539.
 Minicom: 071 821 9812.

The Migraine Trust
45 Great Ormond Street
London WC1N 3HZ
tel.: 071 278 2676

The Samaritans. (S.W. Herts). 45 St. Johns Road, Watford, Herts.
tel.: (0923) 233333

The Spinal Injuries Association (SIA) has launched a telephone service
for spinal cord injured people and their families.   For information,
contact: Adrian Scarfe, SIA, 76 St. James' Lane, London N10 3DF.
tel.: 081 444 2121.
The counselling line is on 081 883 4296.

The Stress Foundation
1 Speldhurst Court
Queens Road
Maidstone
Kent ME16 OJH

The Women's Nationwide Cancer Control Campaign, Suna House,
128-130 Curtain Road, London EC2A 3AR.
tel.: 071 729 2229.

This Book is published by the BOXMOOR OSTEOPATHIC PRESS. I do hope you find it helpful.

The future of OSTEOPATHY depends on the high standard of education and skill instilled in graduates of the 4 year course of osteopathy available at THE BRITISH SCHOOL OF OSTEOPATHY, London.

If you would like to send a contribution to this worthwhile charity please tear off the attached slip and send it with your donation to

"The BSO Appeal"
THE BRITISH SCHOOL OF OSTEOPATHY
1-4 Suffolk Street
LONDON
SW1Y 4HG

(Registered Charity No: 312873)

Cut along this line

115

FROM STRENGTH TO STRENGTH
ORDER FORM

Further copies of this book may be obtained by sending a cheque for the purchase price to:

Brian Cusworth.
9 Northridge Way,
Boxmoor,
Hemel Hempstead,
Herts. HP1 2AE.

Cheques should be crossed and made payable to: **Brian Cusworth**.

Price per book: £4.99 plus £1.00 post and packing.

Please send me ...... copies of
FROM STRENGTH TO STRENGTH.
I enclose a cheque for £ ......

PLEASE ENTER YOUR YOUR DETAILS (IN BLOCK LETTERS) BELOW:

NAME:..

ADDRESS:..

....

....

Postcode:...............................